H.O.P.E. Fitness

Help On Personal Excellence

A Workbook with "YOU" in Mind!

-Jacqueline Corazon

BodyFit H.O.P.E. Publications

H.O.P.E. Fitness by Jacqueline Corazon

ISBN: 978-0615585154

Always consult your physician before beginning any exercise program. This general information is not intended to diagnose any medical condition or to replace your healthcare professional. Consult with your healthcare professional to design an appropriate exercise prescription. If you experience any pain or difficulty with these exercises, stop and consult your healthcare provider.

Foreword

I met Jacqueline while living in Boston when my husband was earning his MPA from Harvard University. Desperate to lose weight, tone, and overall become healthier, I prayed asking God to send help. God answered my prayer by sending me to H.O.P.E. Fitness. Jacqueline inspired me with her personal journey of going from a beauty queen and ballerina, to overweight mother, back to a slim, healthy perfectly built athlete. I could relate to Jacqueline and when I took her classes, they were easy to follow and I felt like "one of the girls." When my husband and I visited New York City for Christmas that year, I knew her classes were working when I didn't get worn out running up and down subway steps, walking for miles around Manhattan and ice skating in the Rockefeller center. I had energy and there was a skip in my step as I treasured walking hand in hand with my Lucas down 5th Avenue perusing the holiday themed store displays. There is something else about Jacqueline you should know. She truly cares about the women who take her classes. She helps everyone individually with their form, and is a natural motivator. If you are a woman like me who is in need of help, Jacqueline can restore your H.O.P.E. for a leaner, fitter, healthier you.

Bethany K. Scanlon
Bestselling Christian Author
-With God, all things are possible!

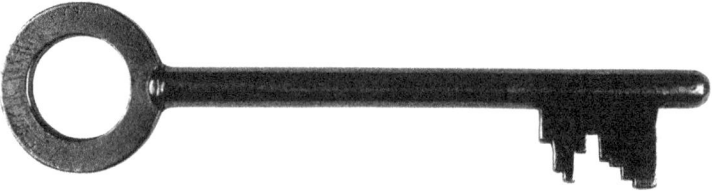

It's about what YOU can do, NOT what others are doing!

TABLE OF CONTENTS

My Experience

I have been in the fitness industry for over 30 years and in great physical and mental health. A former student from the Boston Conservatory of Music and a natural athlete, I have worked hard and creatively over the years to combine dance and fitness for the enjoyment of my students.

I started a career in dance fitness in 1981 while attending the Boston Conservatory of Music as a Dance Major. During my time in school, I was encouraged to enter a Miss Philippines-USA pageant by friends and relatives. The winner of the pageant was to represent the young Filipino women growing up in an America. I won with my talent, intelligence, grace, and beauty. Since winning my title of Miss Philippines USA in 1982, I have been very busy with my career as fitness professional. I have been featured in several fitness magazines such as Shape, Fitness, and Cycling Fitness. I also appeared on several talk shows and fitness segments on major TV networks and danced on various music videos for Kashif, Benjamin Orr, and Semper Fi.

In 1988 I moved to L.A. to further my career and education at UCLA. Almost immediately after moving to LA, I was asked to be an instructor and trainer for Jane Fonda's fitness studio where my list of students and clients included celebrities such as Sharon Gless, Shirlee Fonda and even Jane herself. I also had a following of students from other fitness studios such as Kevin Bacon, Jean-Claude Van Damme, Paula Abdul, Chynna Phillips, Christy Turlington, and the late Juliete Prowse.

One of my interesting accomplishments as a fitness professional was going to Norway in 1991 to choreograph, produce, and perform in an exercise video that featured Miss World Norway. My most memorable experience was going to the Middle East during Desert Storm War, 1991. In Bahrain, myself and five other fitness professionals implemented a fitness and recreational program for the U.S. troops.

Without a doubt, I find my greatest challenge is being a mother of 3 girls and one boy ages 18, 16, 13, and 9. A full time mom, I own and operate BodyFit, Quincy's most affordable and effective gym since 2003.

I am certified in aerobics, Spinning®, Body Pump®, Kick Boxing, Mat Pilates, Zumba®,Jukari® and hold personal training certifications from UCLA and AFAA. My passion is dance-fitness. My calling is to utilize my dance and fitness expertise to combat health and lifestyle issues that plague this country.

My Story of H.O.P.E.

A model and ballet dancer at a young age, the pressure on me to be thin was excruciating. But it started even before that. Issues with body image always plagued me. Born an American Filipino, I was tall and larger framed than most Filipino girls my age. My Filipino peers always teased me. As a classical ballet dancer I always felt if I were thinner I could be more graceful and lift my leg higher. As a model I felt if I was thinner I could get more jobs. I was always watching my weight.

Memories of my mother's disapproval of my weight just heightened my obsession with weight to the point where I became bulimic. I was consumed by my weight. After I was introduced to fitness while living for a short time in LA in the 80's, I was drawn to teaching aerobics. I was finally happy with my weight and I focused on my well-being. I moved back to Boston and continued my career as an aerobics instructor and fitness model.

I even felt confident enough to compete in a beauty pageant that won me the title Miss Philippines -USA. My hunger to learn more about fitness motivated me to move back to LA once again. Missing my family, I returned to New England. After settling back in Boston, I lost sight of my fitness and health. After a life of being disciplined with my weight I felt I was missing out on something. I began to make poor choices. I stayed out late nightly eating and drinking. My weight crept up almost 40 lbs. As an aerobics instructor, to see myself daily that heavy in the mirror wearing nothing but a thong, tights and sneakers was disturbing! I never lost the weight and instead gained even more after meeting my husband and soon after getting pregnant. Four children later, I longed for my model and dancer size. I struggled to take that extra weight off for 17 years. As a former beauty queen, model, and celebrity fitness trainer, depression took hold when I couldn't get back to my ideal weight. After losing all hope, I chose to create my own program that met my needs, a program that was quick, effective and gentle on my aging body. I soon discovered I was not alone. There were so many other women struggling with their weight, some women only needing to lose a few pounds here and there, however, enough to impact their confidence and self worth.

I created H.O.P.E. H.O.P.E. stands for **Help On Personal Excellence** - a fitness program I designed with YOU in mind. This is not written for the women who are 20-something with rock-hard bodies, athletically fit with no injuries, and all the time in the world. Such women can also benefit from this book, but it was written for *you* who I believe, with my help, can lose the weight you have been struggling with, whether it's 5 lbs. or 105 lbs. My approach is safe, progressive, time efficient and non-intimidating. I have the knowledge and the experience. My thirty years of working closely with women, has brought me the wisdom and vision to create this workbook. I will address issues that only concern you. You do not need a college degree in physiology and biomechanics to understand H.O.P.E. Fitness. I was fortunate to have a fitness background from UCLA and 30 years experience in the health and fitness industry to help me win my weight battle. I fought it alone, but now you don't have to! Remember, I was YOU!

PHOTO ALBUM

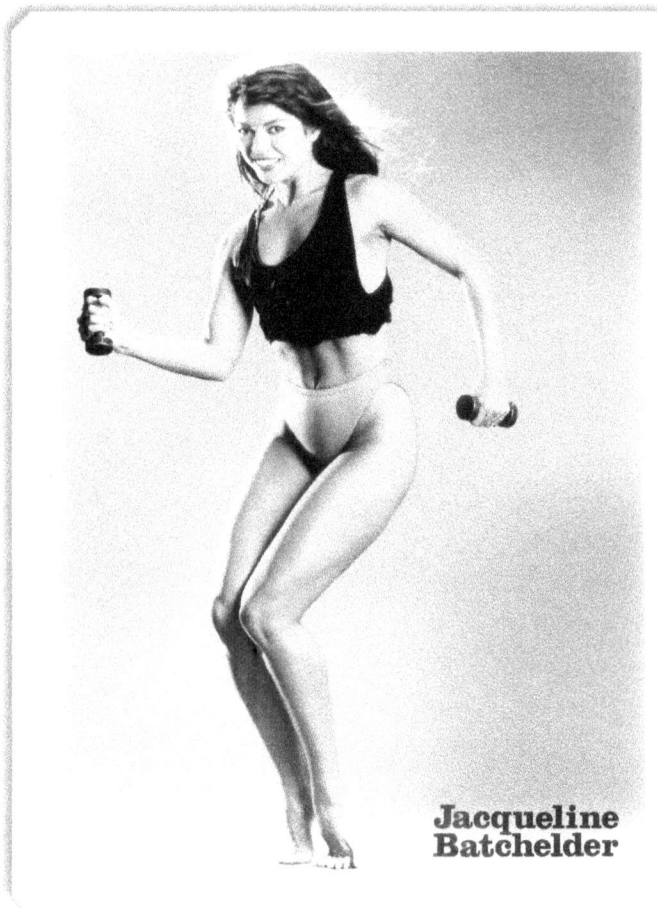

Jacqueline
Batchelder

This is me before marriage and children!

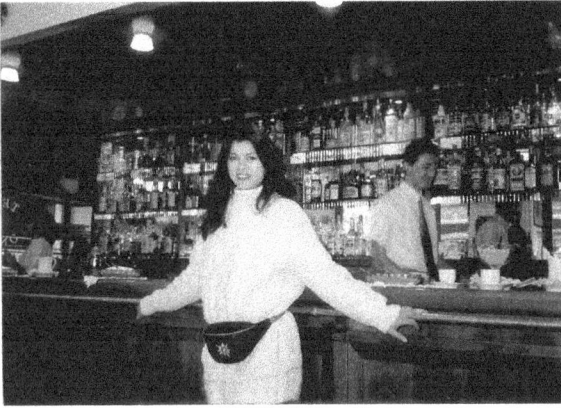

This is me falling in love and enjoying comfort foods!

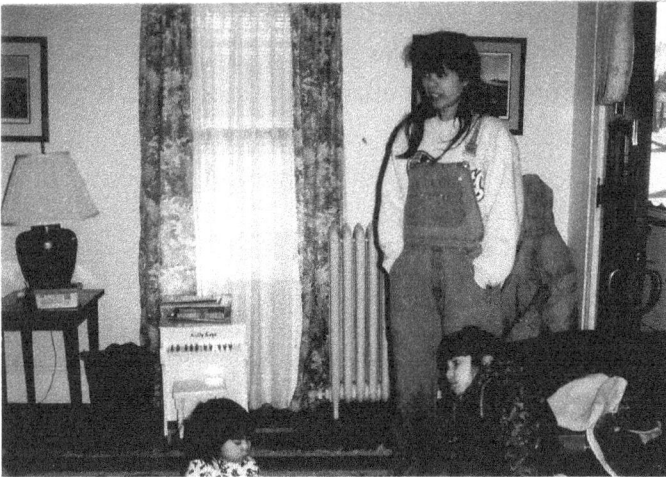

After kids with no time for myself!

Let's get your H.O.P.E. back...

If you could improve your health, tone and sculpt your body, develop better posture, increase your energy in just 30 minutes a day, would you be willing to commit to a 12-week program? If so, this is the best fitness tool you will ever purchase.

H.O.P.E. Fitness was not written to tell you what I know, it's to empower you with information that will help you achieve personal excellence with fitness and conscious eating. Exercises will be explained in language you can understand. A simple exercise routine will give you a sense of accomplishment and a feeling of success. Oh yes...you'll be a few dress sizes smaller. Enjoy your personal fitness journey and discover how great you will look and feel after just 12-weeks.

Before you embark on this personal H.O.P.E. fitness program, you must plan your journey. Like a road trip you must have a map (your H.O.P.E. Fitness Workbook), plan your stops (workout/rest days), pace yourself (measure your accomplishment weekly), and determine when (goal date) you want to reach your goal (total weight loss or dress size you want to achieve).

I am just scratching the surface of fitness with you. You will not find all the answers to your fitness questions in this workbook. However, I am going to address the most common questions asked in my 30+ years of experience in the industry and give you a program that is simple and easy to follow. You must always strive for excellence when it comes to your health and well being. I worked hard on H.O.P.E. Fitness to provide you direction to excellence. Now it's your turn to get to work, using my guidelines to channel your efforts in the most efficient way!

H.O.P.E. Training

The American College of Sports Medicine recommends that all adults need to exercise for 20-60 minutes a day, 3-5 days a week. Your workouts should consist of aerobic activity, resistance training and flexibility work. This is a simple explanation of why aerobic fitness is important and how you can achieve it. Aerobic activity should raise the heart rate (pulse) between 55%-90% of the Maximum Heart Rate. Your maximum heart rate (MHR) can be estimated by subtracting your age from 220. Multiply the MHR by 55% to 90% (Intensity) =Target Heart Rate (THR).

Health related benefits from exercising are (to name a few): lower resting heart rate, improved bone density, lower blood pressure, lower stress level and depression, change in fat and lean muscle ratio, and improved self image and self esteem.

Calculate your training zone range:

220 – AGE = Max Heart Rate

220 - _____ = _____

(Use this figure for MHR in the formula below)

MHR x 55% = Target Heart Rate

_____ x 55% = _____

MHR x 90% = THR

_____ x 90% = _____

(When starting out, train in the 55% range. Advance training is in range of 90%)

If you own a heart rate monitor, the Target Heart Rate calculation is very helpful in monitoring your training heart rate. However, if you don't have one, a simple way to guesstimate how hard your heart is working is by your perceived exertion. Ask yourself how hard you are working on a scale from one to five.

If your answer is:

1 -**Easy** (feeling warm/55%)
2 -**Slightly Hard** (able to have a conversation/65%)
3 -**Hard** (comfortably uncomfortable/75%)
4 -**Very Hard** (breathing heavy/75%)
5 -**Extremely Hard** (breathless/90%)

Let's get started...

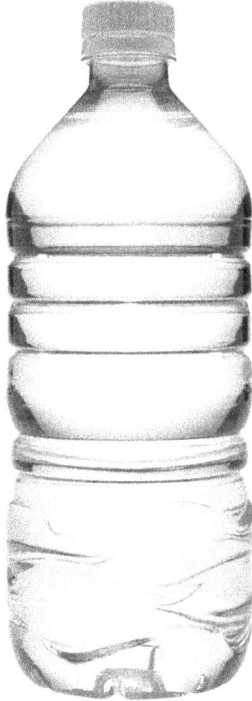

H.O.P.E. Tips: *Always bring water with you when you work out. Drink at least eight glasses of water throughout the day to stay hydrated and healthy!*

H.O.P.E. Fitness

The following exercises are simple to follow, yet effective. H.O.P.E. Fitness encourages weight training because the more muscle you have (lean muscle mass) the higher your resting metabolic rate (RMR). A pound of muscle burns 40 calories a day. If you gain 5 lbs. of muscle, you will increase your calorie burn by 200 calories a day. Additional benefits include higher bone density, increased muscle mass, decreased body fat, increased energy and productivity.

In this workbook, you will find the exercises are named and accompanied with photos (yes, that's me). A description of how you should perform the exercise will be explained and H.O.P.E. Tips will be given. You will also find a chart explaining what muscles you are using and the benefits of conditioning those muscles.

All exercises will begin with the H.O.P.E. Ready Posture (pg. 26). For lying down exercises, a brief explanation on form will be given before performing the exercise. **REPETITION** (reps) means the number of times you perform an exercise (example: 12 repetitions of squats). A **SET** is the number of repetitions repeated with rest in between (example: 2 sets of squats would be 12 repetitions followed by rest then another 12 repetitions). The number of **REPETITIONS** of the exercise will be given (usually 12 reps for each exercise) and as you become more fit, you can increase the amounts of **SETS** of the exercise.

Before you begin, you will need several dumbbells and a mat or large beach towel to lie on the floor. You should have water nearby and a clock with a minute hand. Wear something light and comfortable. Wear appropriate footwear like sneakers. Make sure the room you are exercising in is spacious, cool and ventilated. If you want to play music in the background choose music that is fun and motivating.

The general rule of what weight you should start with is this: if you can perform 8-12 reps with good form that weight is appropriate. If you cannot complete 8-12 reps of the exercise without compromising your form, than it is too heavy. However, if you can do more than 15 reps, the weight is too light and you need to increase the weight. You should then increase the weight once you have established **BASE CONDITIONING** (pg. 25). By increasing the weight you will increase strength, lean muscle, decrease body fat and increase resting metabolic rate (see **H.O.P.E. Training & H.O.P.E. Nutrition)**.

Technically, you should train your largest muscle groups first. But for convenience, the routine is designed so that you perform all standing toning exercise first, then continue remaining toning exercises on the floor. The stretching segment will start standing and finish on the floor. I suggest you choose music that is calming and a slower tempo when stretching and cooling down.

For an aerobic workout, move quickly through the sets. However, do not compromise your H.O.P.E. Ready Posture when executing exercises. Slow and controlled movements are best. Accompany your workout with music that motivates you. However, do not try to keep up with a fast beat. It is important you begin your H.O.P.E. Fitness with a rhythmic warm-up. This will elevate your core temperature, pump blood to your muscles and prepare your heart for the workload ahead.

Exercise is your personal journey. You will discover how your body moves and how exercise affects your well being. Exercises in this workbook will be explained in layman's terms. This program is not written in complex fitness terminology, it is written in a language you can understand and easily follow.

Time to get fit...

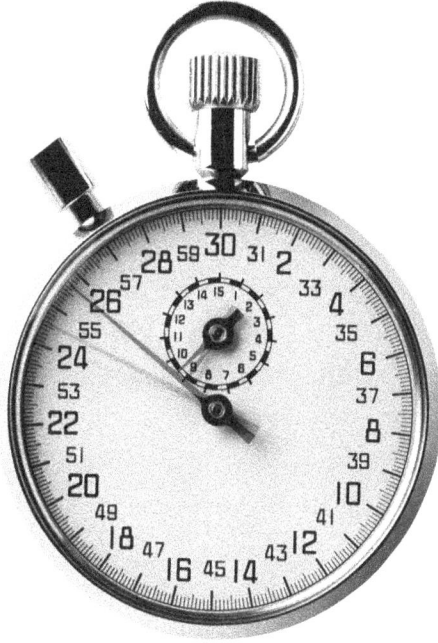

H.O.P.E. Tips: *Wearing a heart rate monitor while you exercise helps you stay within your target heart rate. Some heart rate monitors can also tell you how many calories you are burning!*

Rhythmic Warm-up

Warm up: 5 minutes of rhythmic movements

March for 16 counts

Knee lifts for 16 counts

Side to side lunges 16 counts

Repeat sequence 4 times. If you have a very sedentary lifestyle and/or have never done an aerobic activity, do less repetition and sets. You can increase the sequence of aerobic exercises when your fitness improves. You can also incorporate some dance moves if you like. When you are no longer huffing and puffing after numerous repetitions and sets, you have achieved a higher level of fitness and aerobic capacity. This is called Base Conditioning. Be sure to check your pulse periodically (at the wrist-radial pulse, not neck-carotid artery). Count how many beats per minute. Using your middle and index fingers, feel for the radial artery inside your wrist. You will feel the pulse beating. Do not use your thumb to take the pulse because it has a pulse of its own.

Base Conditioning

Base Conditioning is the level of fitness that you must achieve before progressing to a more aggressive aerobic workout and multiple sets of exercises. Once you have achieved **Base Conditioning**, you can go through the routine with more speed, greater intensity and less rest time between sets. You can also incorporate **Rhythmic Movements** between exercises and increase the number of sets of exercises for a greater aerobic workout. Never compromise your form because you are moving too rapidly or add more repetitions if your joints and muscles are not ready. Poor form and alignment may do more harm than good. Too many repetitions of the same movement may cause prolonged soreness and even tendinitis in the joints if you do not have **BASE CONDITIONING**. One basic rule when training, if the risks outweigh the benefit, don't do it.

H.O.P.E. Ready Posture

H.O.P.E. Ready Posture: Feet firmly on the ground directly below hips. Body weight equally distributed on all corners of both feet. Knee caps lifted, thighs firm, tailbone dropped, chest broad and open, collar bones wide, shoulders down and blades flat against the back, girls up and perky, shining forward and bright:). Maintain a strong and stiff back throughout all movements.

H.O.P.E. Tips: *Don't round your shoulders. Don't collapse the chest. Don't stick your bootie out, or over arch the lower back.*

My Notes:

DO

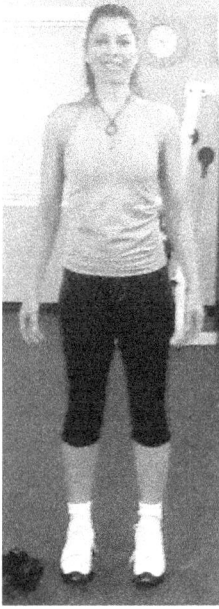

DON'T

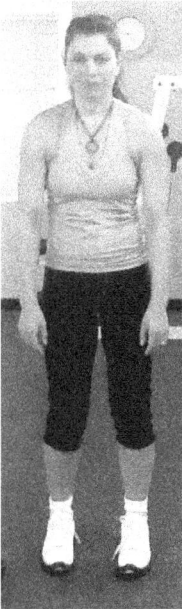 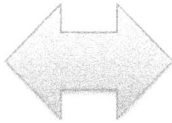 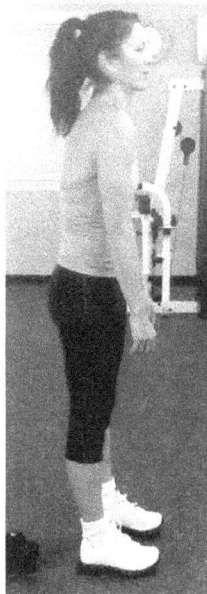

Squats

Standing in H.O.P.E. Ready Posture, feet shoulder width apart, hands behind your head, bend both knees and sit back into heels as if to squat over a toilet in a public restroom. Be sure to keep the Ta-Tas up! To increase intensity, hold dumbbells by your shoulders. Press into heels when coming up from squatting position. Do not include weights until you have completed the twelve-week base conditioning.

H.O.P.E. Tips: *Before you lower into a squat, take a deep breath. Hold the breath so that back is supported by the inflated lungs. Exhale and press weights up when you return to standing position.*

My Notes:

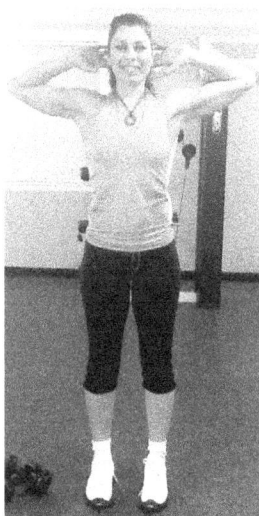
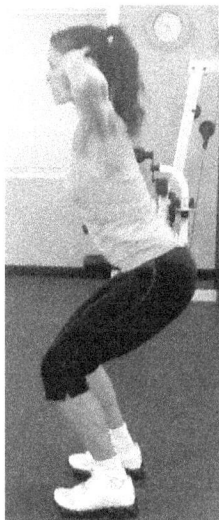
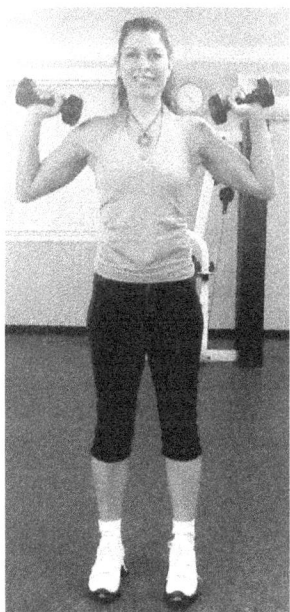
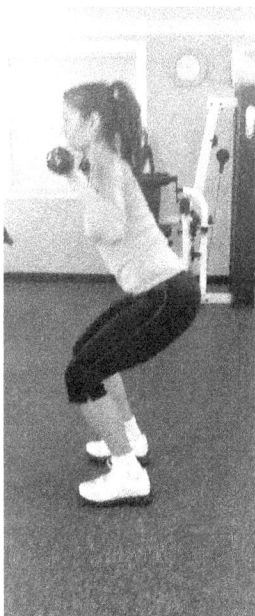

Lunges

Hands behind your head, feet hip width apart, H.O.P.E. Ready Posture. Step back with your left foot directly behind left hip. Landing on the ball of your foot, bend back knee. Front right knee bend will follow. Front right knee should be above ankle and track in line with middle toe in lunge position. Repeat with right leg lunge. Execute 12 repetitions with each leg. To increase intensity, hold dumbbells by your shoulders. Press weights above head when lunging back. Do not use weights until you have completed 12 - week base conditioning.

H.O.P.E. Tips: *When lunging, keep back slightly arched, shoulders back. You should step back far enough so you feel a stretch at the hip flexor and front of thigh of the rear leg. When lunging back without weights, hold your breath for back support. When using weights, exhale when you lunge back and press weights up above your head. Do not allow upper arms to go behind your ears.*

My Notes:

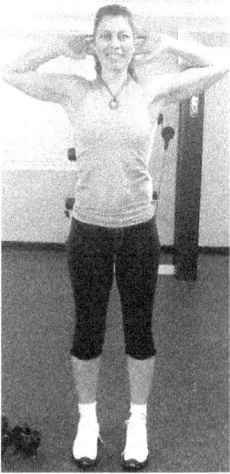
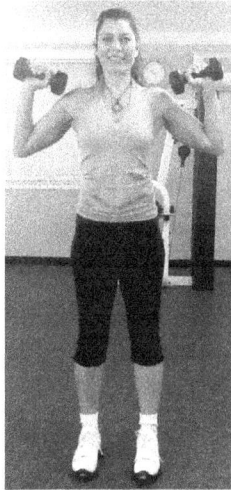
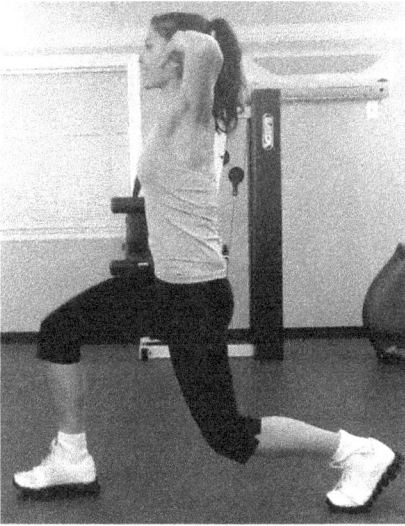
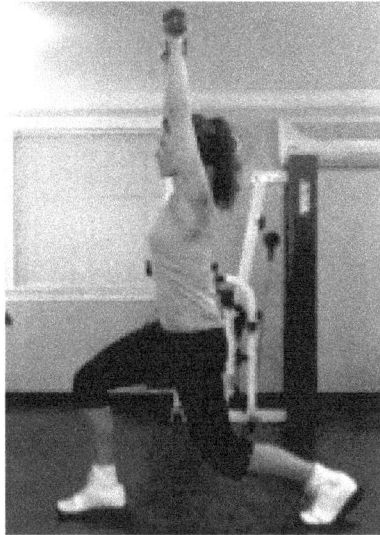

Single Leg Dead Lift

Stand in H.O.P.E. Ready Posture. Bring one leg directly behind hip. Bend forward at the hip. The back leg should lift off the floor as you bend forward. Arms will fall perpendicular to the floor. Stand strong on that one leg. Return to H.O.P.E. ready posture and repeat same leg for a total of 12 repetitions, then switch.

H.O.P.E. Tips: *Abs should be engaged to support forward flexion. Keep back stiff. Do not lock knee of standing leg when flexing forward.*

My Notes:

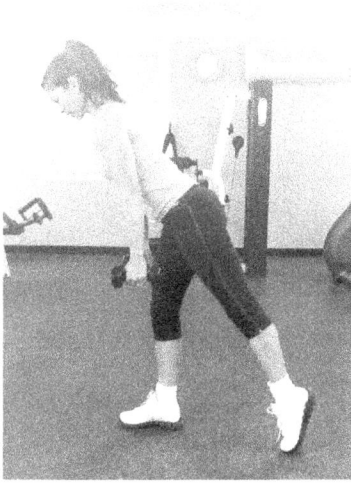

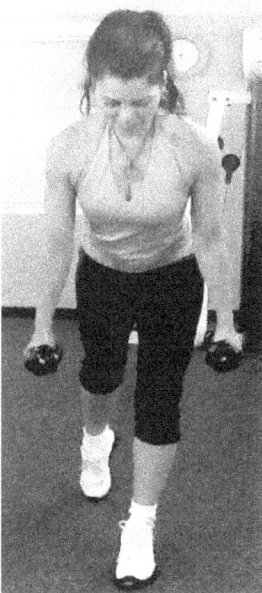

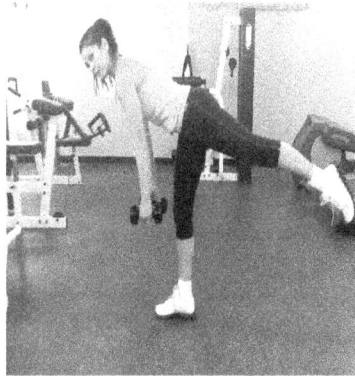

Standing Rows

Start with H.O.P.E. Ready Posture. Bend at the hips until your back is parallel to the floor. Bend your knees if the back of your legs are tight. It is important flexion occurs at the hip, not waist. Raise both elbows upward allowing the elbows to bend to 90 degrees. Keep arms close to the body. Squeeze shoulder blades towards spine at the top.

H.O.P.E. Tip: *Keep abs engaged to support lower back in forward flexion. When raising elbows, keep arms close to body.*

My Notes:

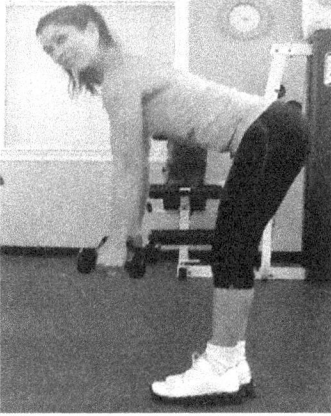

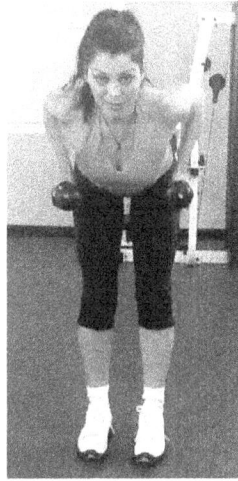

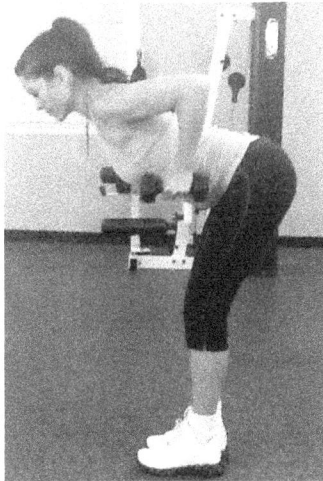

Front Lateral Raise

Stand in H.O.P.E. Ready Posture. Keep back stiff, inside of elbows facing front, soft crease in the elbows, raise both arms on the diagonal to shoulder level only.

H.O.P.E. Tips: *Do not lean back when raising arms. Keep weight equally distributed on all four corners of feet. Do not raise arms above shoulder level. Imaging holding a large steering wheel at 2 O'clock and 10 O'clock at the top of your shoulder lift.*

My Notes:

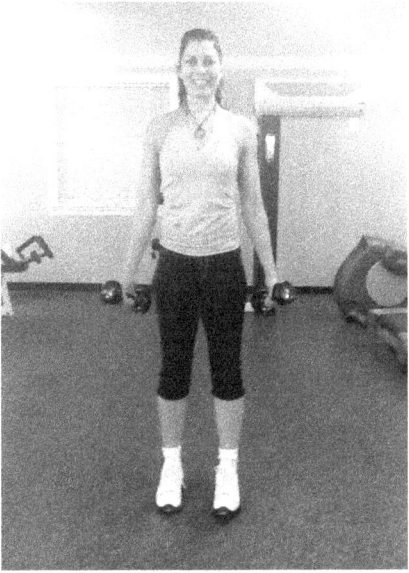

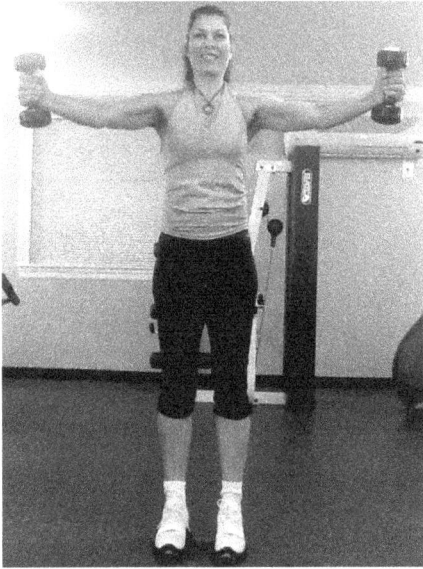

Side Lateral Raise

Standing in wide H.O.P.E. Ready Posture, turn left foot to the diagonal, right foot points forward. Bend left knee and lean your body to the left. Keep both sides of your waist lengthened. Rest your left hand on your left thigh. Right arm is long with a slight crease at the elbow. Elbow facing front, raise right arm to shoulder level. Then lower with control just above the thigh.

H.O.P.E. Tips: *Keep back stiff, chest wide. Do not arch back or lean forward. Raise your arm only to shoulder level. Any higher and you will impinge the shoulder and use your neck muscles (upper trapezius)*

My Notes:

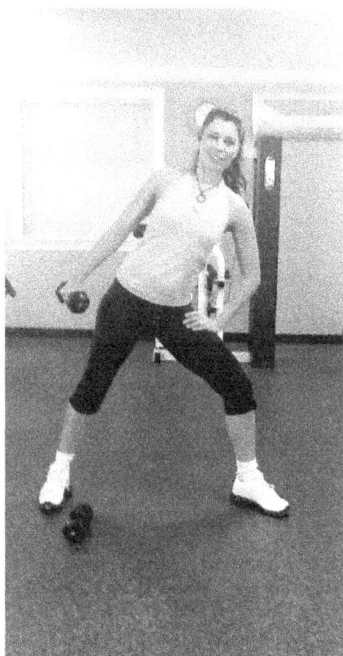

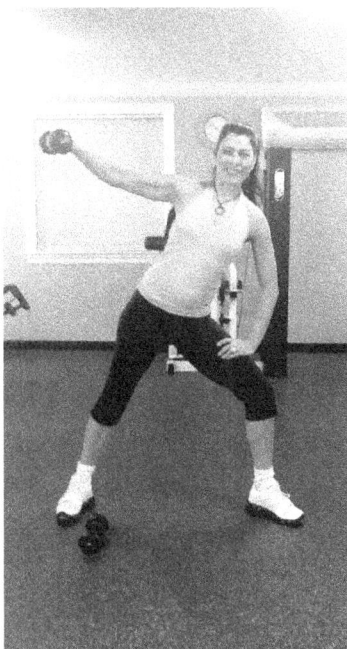

Biceps

Stand in H.O.P.E. Ready Posture. Hold weights next to thigh palms facing forward with crease in elbows. Bend elbows, raise hands to just below the bra line. Shoulder blades remain flat against the back the entire time. Then lower with control.

H.O.P.E. Tips: *Do not lean back when raising arms. Keep body weight equally distributed on all four corners of your feet. Keep wrist stiff and flat.*

My Notes:

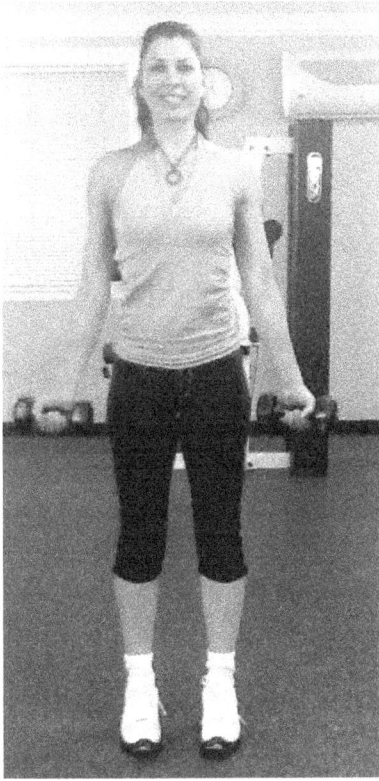

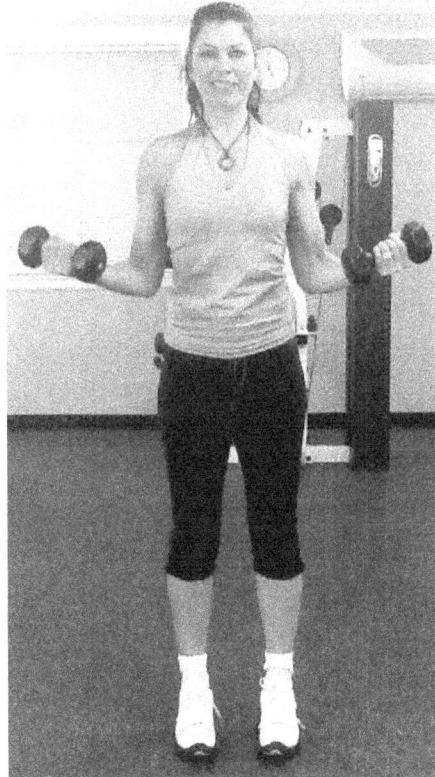

Triceps

Lie on your back with knees bent. Holding a dumbbell in your right hand, place your left hand against the right upper arm for stability. Extend elbow, lifting weight towards the ceiling, then lower hand so that the elbow bends to 90 degrees.

H.O.P.E. Tips: *Do not bend elbows too far or lower hand too close to your head. Do not swing upper arm when extending elbow. Keep your shoulder down.*

My Notes:

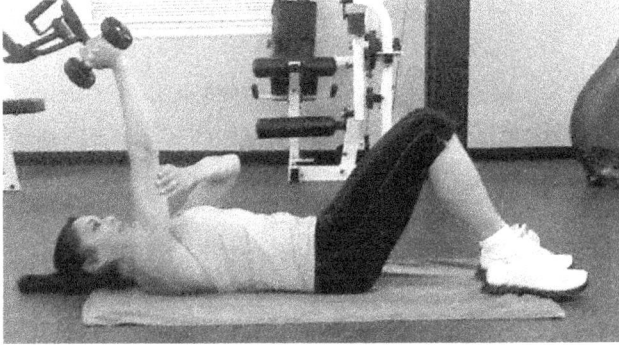

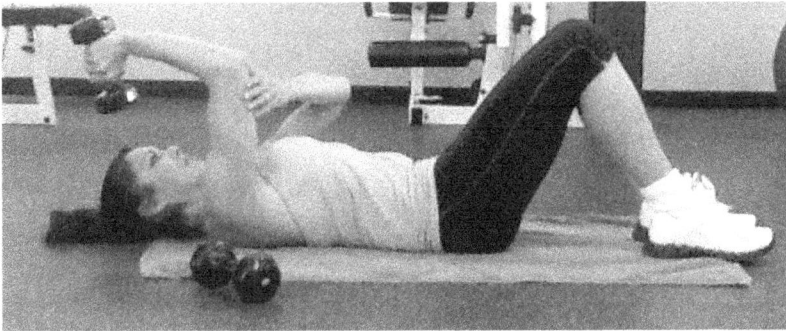

Chest Fly

Lying on your back, bring both legs up to the ceiling, knees slightly bent. When doing floor exercises, it is important to maintain what we call a "neutral spine." That means the spine is neither pressed down to the floor nor arched with space underneath. Bring both arms above your chest. Lower your right arm to the side with a slight crease in your elbow, while the other arm remains perpendicular to the floor. Raise right arm back to center and repeat with left arm. Do this alternating sequence for 12 repetitions.

H.O.P.E. Tips: *Keep abs engaged and upper back flat against the floor. Do not allow opposite shoulder to come off the floor as you lower arm to the side. Do not allow your body to roll towards arm that is lowering to the floor.*

My Notes:

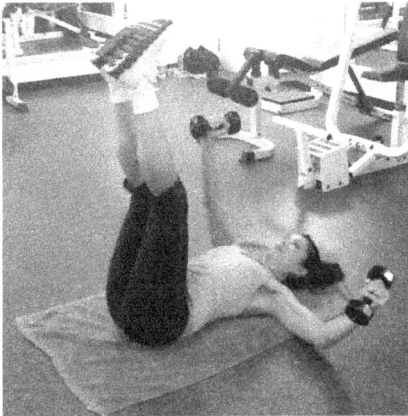

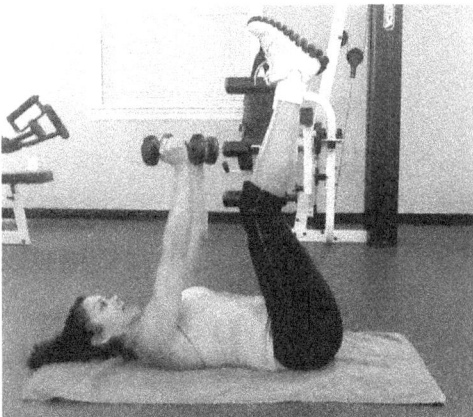

H.O.P.E. Pushups

Lie on your belly, and place hands flat on the floor at nipple level. Slide hands away from body until your wrist are below your elbows. Either on your knees or toes with a stiff body, push off the floor until your elbows are flexed at 90 degrees. Now, raise your body higher until your elbows are extended but not locked. Be sure to keep your shoulder blades down and flat against your back at the top of your push- up. Beginners can do this standing up and pushing against the wall at first, until enough strength is developed to execute push- ups on the floor.

H.O.P.E. Tips: *Do not allow your head to drop. Do not bring your chest lower than your elbows. Do not sway your lower back.*

My Notes:

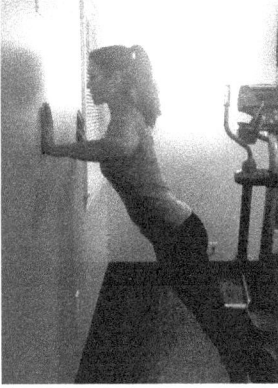

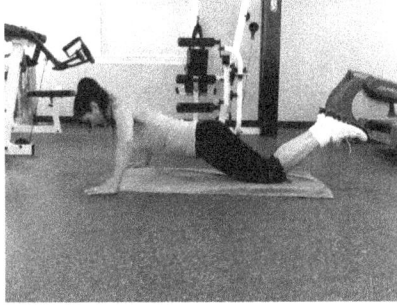

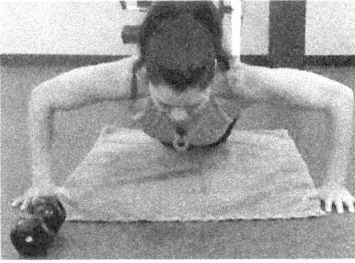

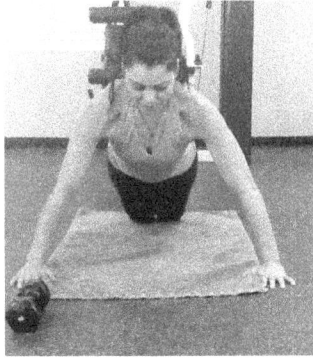

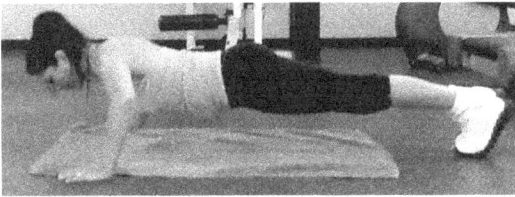

H.O.P.E. Hip Lift

Lie on your back and draw right knee tight to the chest. Left foot should be below knee. Lift hips off the floor and extend left hip, and lower (do not touch your buttocks to the floor when lowering). Do 12 repetitions. Then repeat with other leg.

H.O.P.E. Tips: *Contract your butt muscles when lifting. Do not allow butt to touch floor when lowering between repetitions. Do not tilt your hips.*

My Notes:

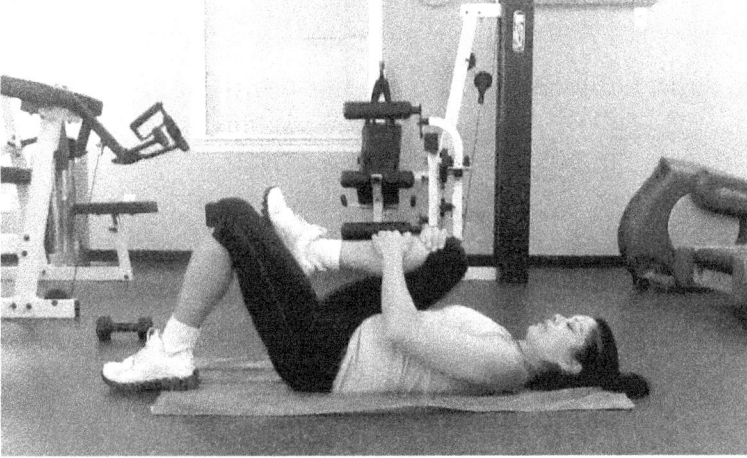

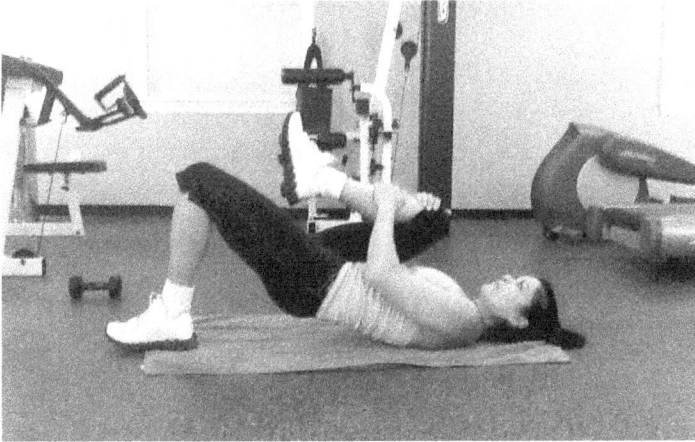

H.O.P.E. Abs

Lie on your back with both knees bent. Raise both knees close to chest, fingers touching shoulders so that your upper back remains flat on the floor. Slowly lower alternating feet towards the floor. Raise head and shoulders off the floor only if you have achieved core strength.

H.O.P.E. Tips: *Draw belly into body, keep shoulders on the floor if you're just starting out. Do not allow back to arch when lowering feet. Keep knees bent at a 90 degree angle when lowering leg towards the floor.*

My Notes:

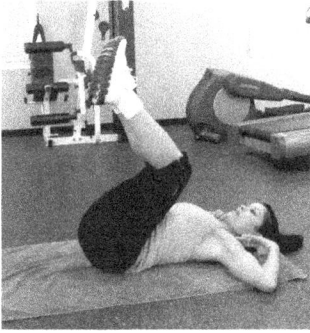

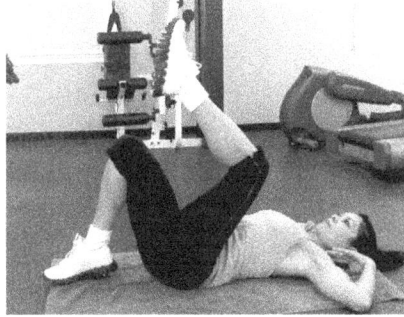

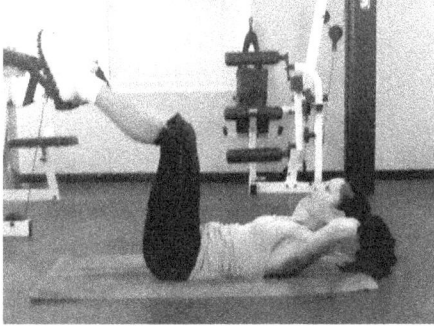

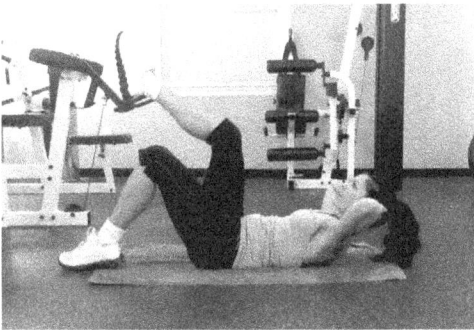

H.O.P.E. Pointer

Start on your hands and knees. Hands below your shoulders, knees under your hips, spine lengthened, pelvis facing floor, belly drawn into the body, eyes focused on the floor. Raise and extend right leg and left arm so they are both parallel and even to the floor. Hold for 10 seconds, then lower. Repeat with other leg and arm. Do alternating sides for 12 repetitions.

H.O.P.E. Tips: *Do not allow back to sway. Keep hips level. Do not allow head to hang. Raise extended arm only to ear level. A straight line should be drawn from the finger tips all the way to the heel of the foot in the air.*

My Notes:

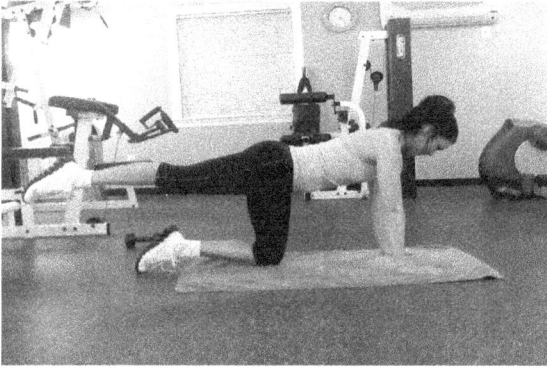

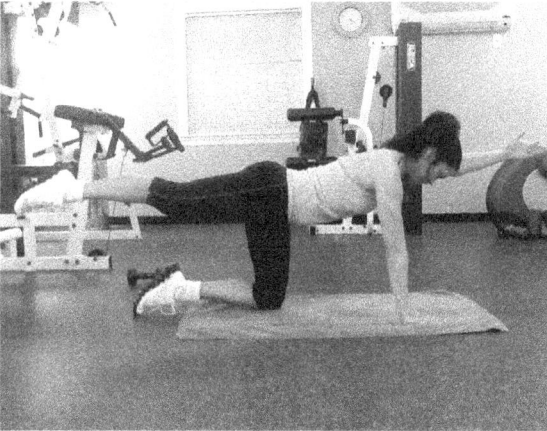

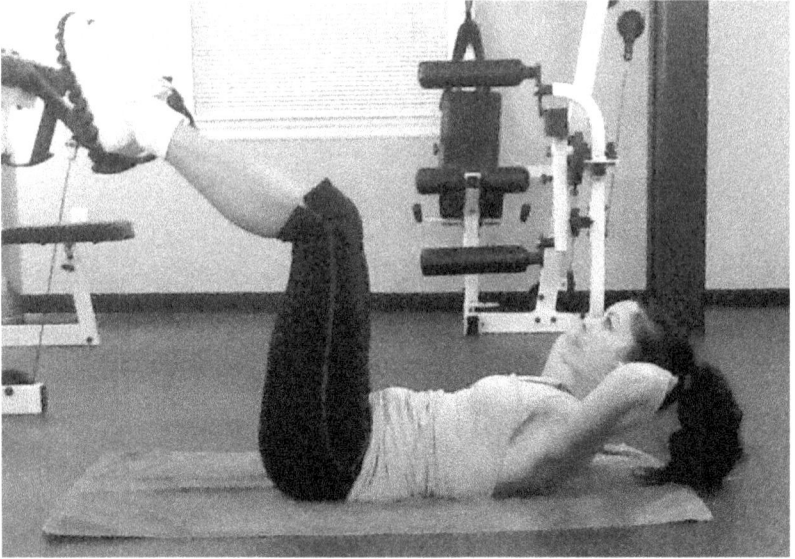

Fit abominable muscles support internal organs and aid in digestion.

H.O.P.E.
Stretches

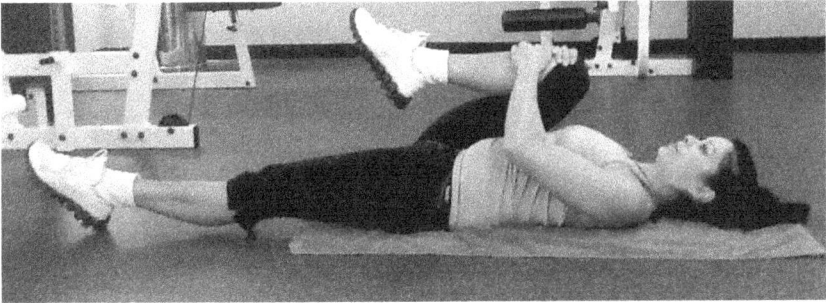

Hamstring Stretch

Standing in H.O.P.E. Ready Posture. Step left foot forward. Bend back knee and pull hips back as if to bow. Shift weight onto right leg. Keep left leg straight. Both hands resting on right thigh. Keep back straight, chest high, abs engaged and back of neck long. Hips and shoulders should be even. Repeat other side.

H.O.P.E. Tips: *Do not bend at the waist. To increase stretch, bend back knee more. To stretch calf, lift toes towards your nose.*

My Notes:

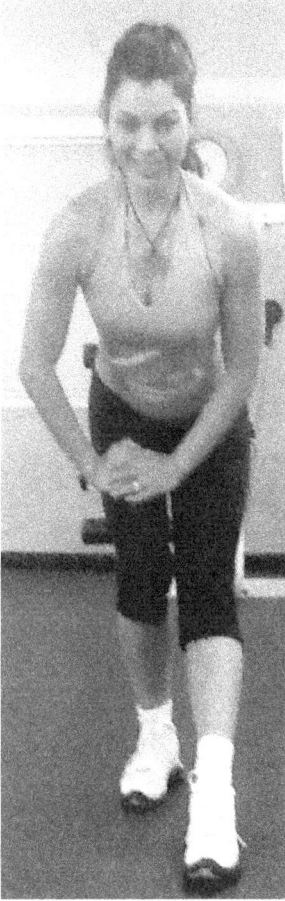

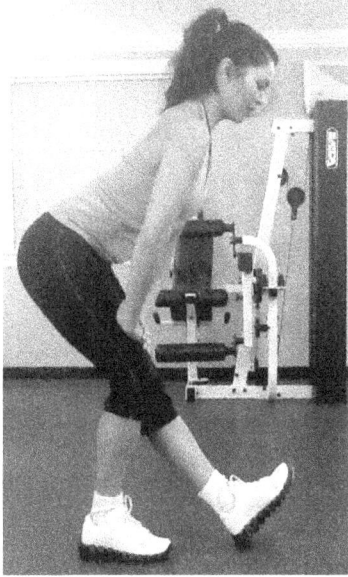

Shoulder Stretch

Standing in H.O.P.E. Ready Posture, bring one arm straight across chest. The other hand will gently hold the lower arm and press arm towards the body. Repeat other side.

H.O.P.E. Tips: *Do not allow shoulders to lift. Do not tug too hard.*

My Notes:

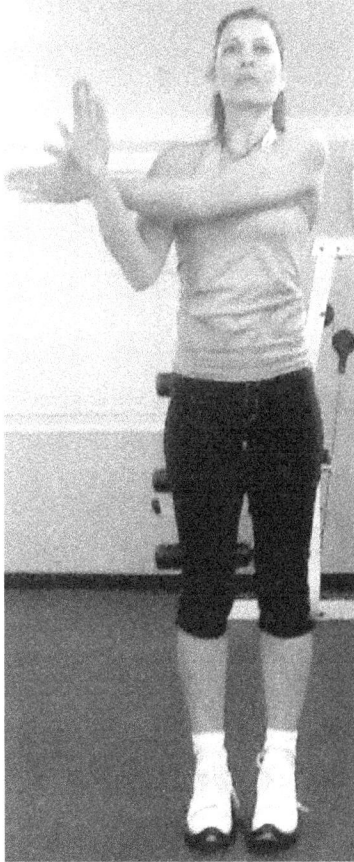

Triceps Stretch

Standing in H.O.P.E. Ready Posture, reach behind your head towards the opposite shoulder with your right hand. With left hand resting above the right elbow, gentle pull elbow inward. Repeat other side.

H.O.P.E. Tips: *Do not pull on the elbows too far. Keep shoulders down.*

My Notes:

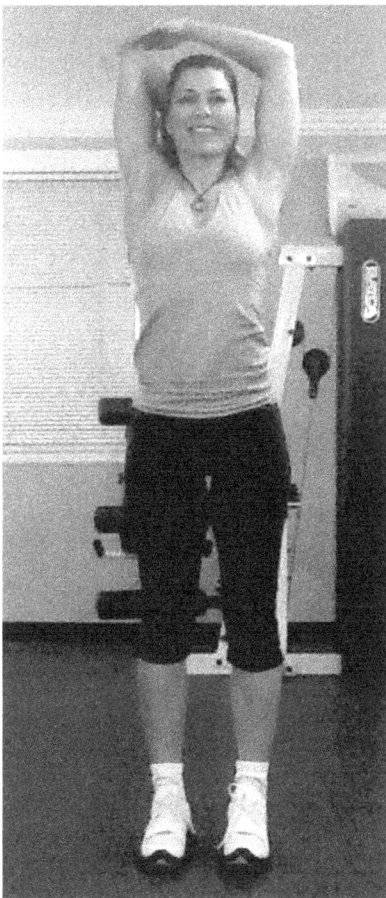
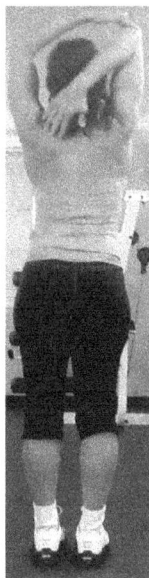

Lower Back Stretch

Lie on your back with both knees bent and feet flat on the floor. Raise your right arm above your head and reach left hand with palms facing up directly to your side at shoulder level. Slowly lower both knees to your left. Repeat other side.

H.O.P.E. Tips: *Keep both shoulders down. Keep knees together. Focus forward. Exhale as you roll knees to the side. Inhale when raising knees back to center.*

My Notes:

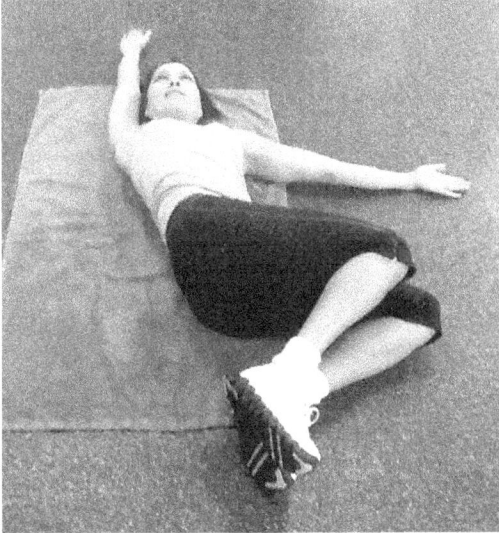

Cat Stretch

On all fours, hands under shoulders, knees underneath hips, draw your abs in and round out your back. Tuck your chin and tailbone under. Release back and return to neutral spine. Repeat other side.

H.O.P.E. Tips: *Exhale when rounding out the back. Inhale when you return to neutral spine.*

My Notes:

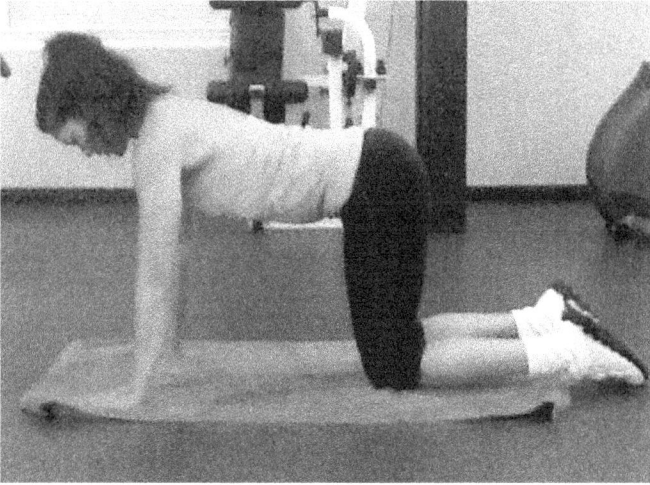

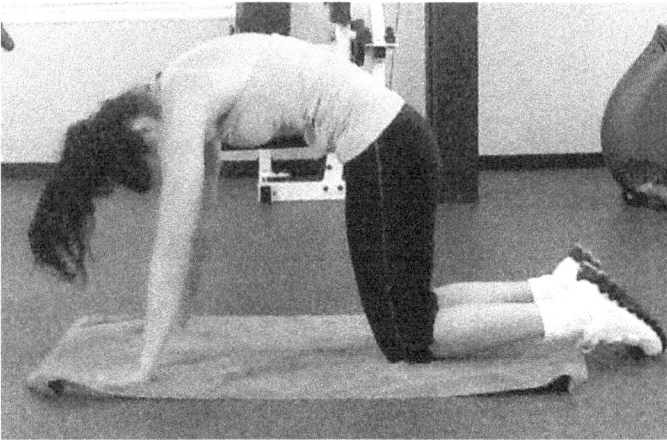

Hip and Groin Stretch

Lie on your back, bend both knees. Cross right ankle above left thigh. Reach the right hand behind the left thigh on the inside, and the left hand behind the left thigh on the outside and interlace the fingers. Gently pull left thigh towards body. Switch legs. Repeat other side.

H.O.P.E. Tips: *Keep back flat against the floor. Tailbone pointing down, lengthen back of the neck. Do not lift shoulders.*

My Notes:

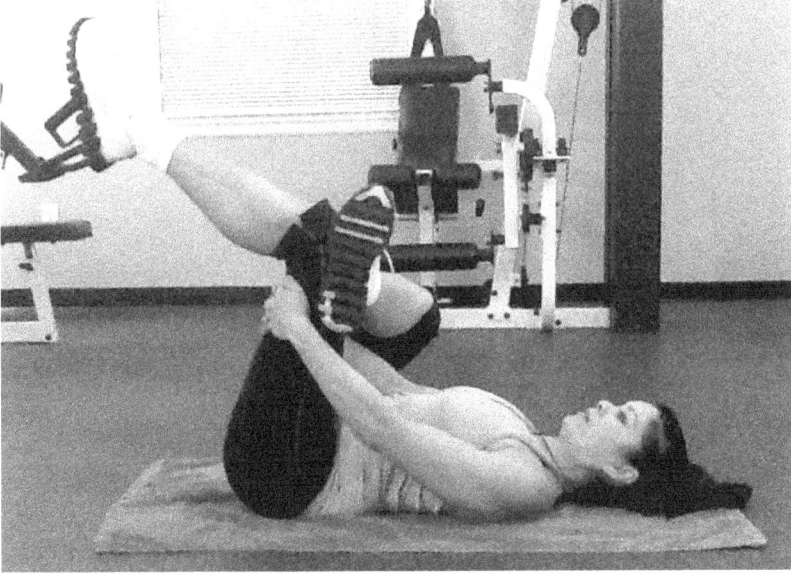

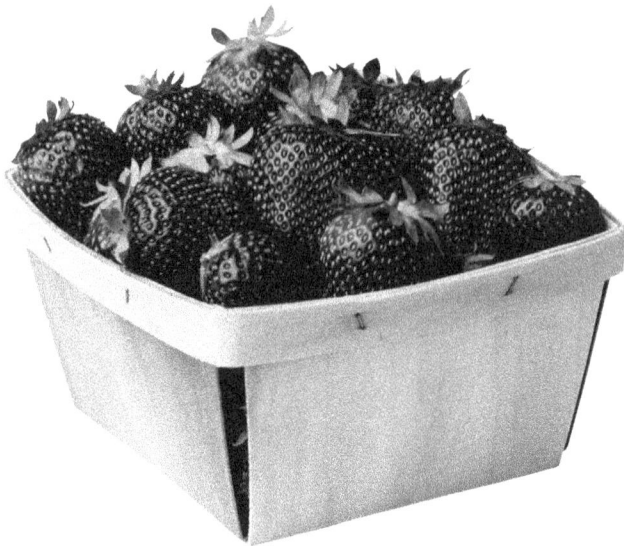

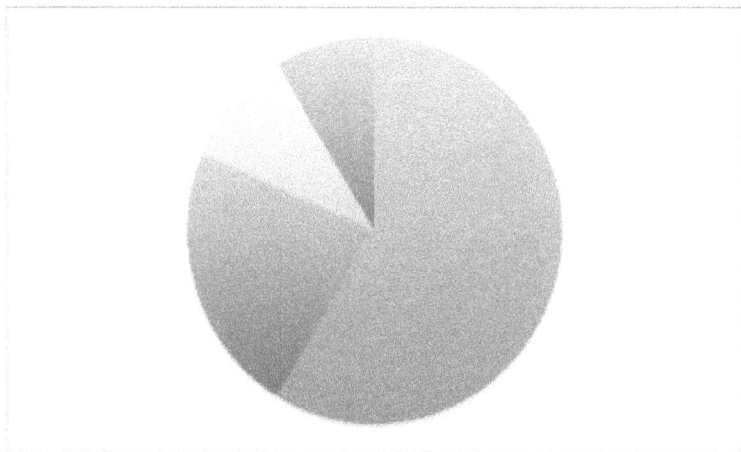

H.O.P.E. Pie Chart:

55-60% Carbohydrates
12-15% Protein
25-30% Fat
Less than 10% Saturated Fat

H.O.P.E. Nutrition

Exercise alone is not enough. One must modify eating behavior. What diet should you follow? None (unless it's a diet recommended by a registered dietitian). Whenever you restrict caloric intake you will see weight loss immediately over a short period of time. Unfortunately, rapid weight loss in the first few weeks of dieting is mostly water loss and may actually cause a lower Resting Metabolic Rate eventually (RMR -the rate in which your body burns calories).

The safest diet is one that meets all your nutritional requirements. Weight loss should not be more than 2 lbs. a week. The American Dietetic Association recommends that your diet should consist of 55-60% carbohydrates, 12-15% protein, 25-30% fat, and <10% saturated fat. Visualize your dinner plate (breakfast/lunch/dinner); it should consist of complex carbohydrates the size of a baseball, protein no larger than a hockey puck, fat total no more than the size of a Ping-Pong ball (sour cream, butter, cheese, etc.). Need another visual? How about a pie graph? Divide a pie into 10 equal parts. Carbs should be 6 parts, protein 1.5 parts, total fat 3 parts, and .5 part saturated fat.

If you do not have a medical condition requiring the advice or help of a registered dietitian, you can determine your needed caloric intake according to your activity level and current weight. You can lose weight safely, prevent your RMR from dropping and change your eating habits permanently just by following these simple tips and suggestions. Remember not only do you want to look good, you want to be healthier and feel good!

In order to become healthier and have lots of energy through out the day, you must make correct food choices. Let's first learn how to read food labels. Most store bought foods today provide the number of carbs, protein, and fat. One gram of carbohydrates is 4 calories. One gram of protein is 4 calories and one gram of fat is 9 calories. A snack item equaling 100 calories that has 4 grams of fat, 2 grams of protein, and 16 grams of carbs would be a great snack. The total calories from this snack are mostly from carbs and your total fat calories are just a little over 30%.

When a snack has over 50% of fat calories, skip that snack and opt for something with less fat and higher nutritional value. Try to avoid foods with empty calories. Foods with empty calories are foods high in fat and sugar and have no nutritional value.

Now that you have some knowledge about reading labels, let's begin to calculate how many calories you are allocated per day in order to lose weight.

Let's start by determining your caloric requirement for your current weight. Your caloric requirement is the amount of calories your body needs just for bodily function. This is called your Resting Metabolic Rate (RMR), such as breathing, eating, digestion, sleeping, reading this workbook, etc.

In order to calculate your RMR, lets calculate your weight in kilograms. To do this, take your weight in lbs. and multiply by .45. Each kilogram requires 24 cal/day, so multiply your weight in kilograms by 24 to get your basic daily caloric needs. Example: 150 lbs. x .45= 67.5 kg x 24 cal/day = 1,620 cal/day. If you are an active person you may require more calories. Add 50% more to your total cal/day (50% x 1,620= 810) 1,620 + 810= 2,430 cal/ day. So, an active person (one who does hard labor or is physically active) can eat up to 2,430 cal/day and this will maintain the person's weight. Add 40% for a moderately active lifestyle. Add 30% if you do light activity daily (above sedentary lifestyle).

Now, if you want to lose approximately 2 lbs. a week, you must be in a caloric deficit of at least 3,500 calories a week. That's a lot! Hence the reason why losing over 2 lbs. a week, realistically, can't all be from fat. How does one be in a deficit of 3,500 calories a week? Well, let's think daily deficit. You can eat 500 calories less a day for 7 days or engage in your H.O.P.E. fitness that burns up to 250 calories an hour and eat 250 calories less daily for 7 days.

Example: Caloric Requirement for 150 lb. person

	RMR	30%	40%	50%
150 lbs.	1620 cal/day	2106 cal/day	2268 cal/day	2430 cal/day

Calculate your RMR

(RMR/caloric requirement for weight maintenance)

Your weight in kilograms

_____ x .45 = _____ weight in kg

_____ (weight in kg) x 24 calories = _____ cal/day

Active person: Add 50% more calories to get your RMR.

Moderately active: Add 40% more calories to get your RMR.

Lightly active: Add 30% more calories to get your RMR.

Once you have determined your caloric need, subtract 500 calories from your calculated RMR daily, in order to lose at least two pounds a week.

Now, let's start your food journal. Buy a small notebook or download an App to track your caloric intake. There are charts at the end of this workbook to track your progress.

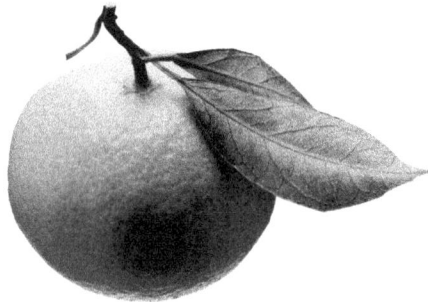

H.O.P.E. Tips for food Choices

Skip the yolk. Eat whites of eggs.

When buying bread, choose a loaf that's heavy. If it feels light, there's very little fiber. Use one slice of bread instead of two. Especially buns. Unless you want it on *your* buns.

Skip the high caloric coffee drinks. Total empty calories! Muffins and bagels are made so much larger these days. Skip it and have English muffins instead.

Skip the instant oatmeal and eat the real deal. Irish oatmeal is best.

Limit alcohol intake. Alcohol consumption encourages poor food choices.

At parties stay away from the buffet table, mingle instead:)

Limit red meat.

Treat yourself on occasion with something sweet so that you won't feel deprived and end up binging anyway.

Skip the bread and butter at the restaurant. Tell the waiter ahead of time so you won't be tempted.

Order a few low calorie appetizers instead of a main course. Food portions today are larger than ever!

When ordering a salad, always ask for dressing on the side. This way you control the amount. Restaurants tend to over do it. Salad dressings can be very high in fat calories.

Avoid fried foods. Have it grilled instead

Skip the chips. It's impossible to have just a few! Empty calories! Skip any processed foods if one of the ingredients is spelled with the letter **X** in (maltodeXtrin, Xamthan gum, deXtrose) and you can't pronounce it. If a food item has an ingredient that ends in **"ose"** or **"oritol"** it is a hidden sugar and you probably should limit if not eliminate that food item. Before you choose a food think about how many times it has been altered before reaching your plate. Can you really identify what is in it? The closer the food is to its natural origin, the better for you! A banana comes from a tree. Chips came from a potato, but you can't be sure how many times it was processed before it ended up in the bag!

In closing, I hope you found this H.O.P.E. Fitness workbook helpful, easy to follow and motivating. I have dedicated my life helping those that have lost all hope gain a healthy and more fit body. If I brought hope to you, then I feel truly blessed. I feel privileged to share my commitment to fitness with you. Best wishes and success on your fitness journey. Here's to your personal excellence!

Yours in health and fitness,

-Jacqueline Corazon

H.O.P.E. Exercise Review

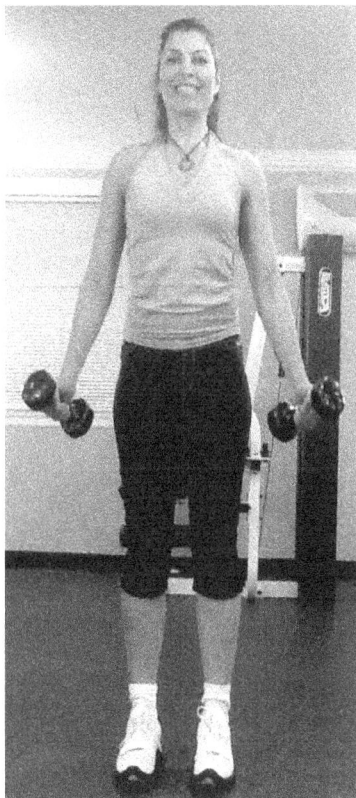

Start with a smile in
H.O.P.E. Ready Posture!

EXERCISE	Starting Position	Movement Cue	Muscle Used	Reps/sets	Notes
H.O.P.E. Ready Posture	Stand with feet hip width apart. Shoulders back, chest high, abs engaged. Back stiff.	No movement. Brace yourself from being pushed or shoved. Feel like a tree with roots grounded.	Abs, back (erector spinae), all muscles of the legs (quads,calfs, hamstring), butt (gluteus).	Begin all standing exercise in H.O.P.E. Ready Posture.	Weight equally distributed on both feet. Pull up on thigh muscles and lift knee caps. Wide across the collar bone.
Squats	H.O.P.E. Ready Posture. Hands behind the head or hand held weights held by the shoulders.	Sit back as if to use a toilet in a public restroom. Keep head up as if to balance a book on top of your head.	Butt muscles (gluteus), abs, back muscles (erector spinae), shoulders (shoulders- if using weights), all the muscles of the legs and feet.	Start with 8-12 reps. Work up to 2 sets.	Do not arch back. Rock body weight towards heels when sitting back. Keep shoulders back, abs engaged. Do not go any lower if you begin to feel it in the knees.

Lunges	H.O.P.E. Ready Posture. Hands behind the head or hand held weights held by the shoulders.	Step back as if to kneel down on back knee. Both knees will bend. You should feel a stretch on the front of the back hip as you step back.	Butt muscles, Inner and outer thigh muscle, shoulders (if using weights), all the muscles of the legs and feet.	Start with 8-12 reps with each leg. Work up to 2 sets.	Shoulders above hips the entire time. Front knee should be above the ankle. Back heel should be off the floor.
Single Leg Dead Lift	H.O.P.E. Ready Posture. Hold hand held weights next to thigh.	Tilt forward at the hip. As head moves towards the floor, foot lifts behind. You will look like a like a see-saw balancing on the standing leg. Keep both hips forward.	Butt muscles (gluteus), back of the standing leg (hamstrings), calf, back and abs	Start with 8-12 reps with each leg. Work up to 2 sets.	Keep body stiff. Bend forward at the hips not the waist. Pull up on the standing leg, lift knee cap and pull up on the thigh. Focus on an object to help with balance.

Standing Rows	H.O.P.E. Ready Posture. Bend forward at the hip with arms hanging from the shoulders towards the floor holding dumbbells in each hand.	Using your butt muscles to support you in this forward flexion, lift both weights towards waist line squeezing shoulder blades.	Butt (gluteus), back of the legs (hamstrings), back muscles (lats, upper trapezius), back of the shoulder(rear deltoids), biceps	Start with 8-12 reps. Work up to 3 sets	Focus on the lats doing the work and not the biceps. Keep elbows close to the body, flexion at the hip, back stiff, back of the neck extended.
Front Lateral Raise	H.O.P.E. Ready Posture. Holding weights by thighs, palms facing front, soft crease in the elbow.	Hold hands 2 o'clock and 10 o'clock, as if holding a large steering wheel.	Front of the shoulder muscles (frontal deltoids).	Start with 8-12 reps. Work up to 3 sets	Do not lean back when raising your arms. Keep your body weight equally distributed on all corners of your feet.

Side Lateral Raise	H.O.P.E. Ready Posture. Bend your left knee and lean to the left. Lowering left shoulder towards the floor. Holding a dumbbell in right hand above the thigh.	Pretend your back is leaning against the wall. Stay flat across your back. Raise weight to shoulder level as if to air out your armpits.	Side of the shoulder muscle (medial deltoids).	Start with 8-12 reps with each arm. Work up to 3 sets.	Do not lean forward or back with shoulders. With a soft crease in the elbow, inside of elbow should face front.
Bicep Curl	H.O.P.E. Ready Posture. Hold hand held weights next to thigh palms facing forward with crease in elbows.	Hold arms in front of body as if to lift a tray. Raise both hands up just below the bra line.	Biceps, Shoulder muscles for upper arm stabilization.	Start with 8-12 reps. Work up to 3 sets.	Shoulder blades remain flat against the back the entire time. Keep weight equally distributed on all four corners of your feet. Keep wrist stiff and flat.

79

Tricep Extension	Lie on your back with knees bent. Holding a dumbbell in your right and, placing your left hand against the right upper arm for stability.	Extend elbow as if to hammer the ceiling. Contract the back of the upper arm.	Muscles in the back of your upper arm (triceps).	Start with 8-12 reps with each arm. Work up to 3 sets.	Do not swing upper arm when extending elbow. Do not life weight with the shoulder. Do not lower hand too close to your head.

EXERCISE Floor Work	Starting Position	Movement Cue	Muscle Used	Reps/ Sets	Notes
One Arm Fly	Lie on your back with both legs up and both arms above chest with weights in hand.	Open one arm out to the side as if to open a cabinet door on your back. Keep the other arm straight up towards the ceiling.	Chest muscles (pectoral), shoulder muscles (frontal deltoids), and abs.	Start with 8- 12 reps alternating arms. Work up to 3 sets.	Do not allow your body to roll towards the arm lowering. Keep both shoulder blades flat against the floor the entire time. Keep butt flat on the floor.
Push Ups	Lie on your belly, chest between hands, wrist below elbows. Start either on your knees or on your toes.	Lower your chest about a fist size distance from the floor. Keep your nose facing down as if to smell the floor.	Chest muscles (pectoral), shoulders (frontal deltoids) back of the upper arms (triceps), and abs.	Start with 8-12 reps. Work up to 3 sets.	Do not allow your shoulders to go below elbows. Do not allow your back to sway.
Hip Lift	Lie on your back. Draw right knee into chest. Hold on to knee. Dig left heel into the floor.	Squeeze butt muscles as if it were a sponge as you raise your butt up.	Butt (gluteus) and muscles of back of thing (hamstring).	Start with 8-12 reps with each leg. Work up to 3 sets.	Don't tilt pelvis, use lower back muscles. Between reps. don't rest butt on floor. Press body weight into heel when raising your butt.

81

Abs	Lie on your back with both knees bent.	Raise both knees close to chest, fingers touching shoulders so that your upper back remains flat on the floor.	Abs (rectus abdominal), transverse, internal and external obliques)	30-50 reps alternate legs. 2-3 sets.	Keep hips stable on the floor. Draw belly in. To increase intensity, lift shoulders off the floor and rotate upper body towards opposite knee that is lifting towards chest.
Pointer	Start on your hands and knees. Hands below your shoulders, knees under your hips.	Spine lengthened, pelvis facing floor, belly drawn into the body, eyes focused on the floor.	Back muscle (erector spinae),butt (gluteus), abs.	Hold for 10 seconds. Repeat with other leg and arm. Alternate sides 12 reps	Do not allow back to sway. Raise arms only the height of ears. Do not lock elbow. Keep back of the neck long.

82

EXERCISE	Starting Position	Movement Cue	Muscle Used	Reps and Sets	Notes
Standing Stretches					
Hamstring Stretch	H.O.P.E. Ready Posture. Bring left leg forward. Bend at the hip. Shift weight onto right leg and bend knee. Keep left leg straight. Both hands resting on right thigh.	Bring hips back as if to bow. Keep your back long and stiff.	Back of the legs (hamstring), calf and lower back.	Hold stretch for 10-20 seconds. Switch legs, hold for 10-20 seconds.	Bend at the hip not waist. Pull hips back evenly. Do not lock front knee. Keep shoulders even.
Shoulder Stretch	Standing in H.O.P.E. Ready Posture, bring one arm straight across chest. The other hand will gently hold the lower arm.	Reach arm across your body as if to shake someone's hand to the other side of you. Then use other hand to press arm closer to body.	Side of shoulder (medial deltoids)	Hold stretch for 10 seconds then switch arms.	Do not allow shoulders to rise up.

EXERCISE	Starting Position	Movement Cue	Muscle Used	Reps and Sets	Notes
Tricep Stretch	Standing in H.O.P.E., reach right hand behind your head towards opposite shoulder blade. With your left hand resting above the right elbow.	Reach hand behind your head as if to scratch your opposite shoulder blade. With the other hand gently pull elbow inward.	Back of the upper arm (triceps) and shoulders	Hold stretch for 10-20 seconds.	Keep shoulders down.
Floor Stretches					
Cat Stretch	All on fours, hands under shoulders, knees underneath hips.	Draw belly into body and round your back like an angry cat. Tuck chin under. Then release back to neutral spine.	Upper back between shoulder blades (traps,rhomboids), lower back.	Hold stretch for 5-10 seconds and return to start position. Do 3-5 reps.	Exhale as you round your back. Inhale when you extend the spine.

84

EXERCISE	Starting Position	Movement Cue	Muscle Used	Reps and Sets	Notes
Hip/Hamstring Stretch	Lie on your back with both legs extended.	Draw right knee in towards body. Keep left leg extended and the back of that knee pressed against the floor.	Butt and back of thigh of bent knee. Front of thigh (quads and hip flexor) of extended leg. Lower back.	Hold for 30 seconds and repeat with other leg.	Exhale as you stretch. Lengthen the lower back towards the floor as you pull the knee closer to your body.
Hip and Groin Stretch	Lie on your back. Cross right ankle above left thigh. Reach right hand behind left thigh while the left hand reaches outside the left thigh. Lace fingers behind left thigh.	Pull thigh towards chest like you are folding body in half by the hip.	Butt (gluteus), inner thigh (abductors), lower back.	Hold stretch for 30 seconds then switch legs.	Keep shoulders, butt and back flat against the floor.

H.O.P.E. Agreement

I _____, accept help on achieving personal excellence by following this 12-week H.O.P.E. Fitness Program. I will accomplish my weight loss of _____lbs. by _____. I will follow the H.O.P.E. Fitness program at least _____ times a week no matter what! I want to lose this weight because_____

_____

_____

_____. Besides the reward of feeling great about myself, I plan on rewarding myself with

_____

_____

_____

_____.

H.O.P.E. _____
(Signature)

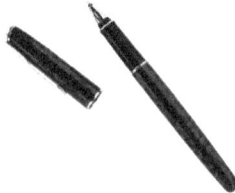

86

Letters of Recommendation

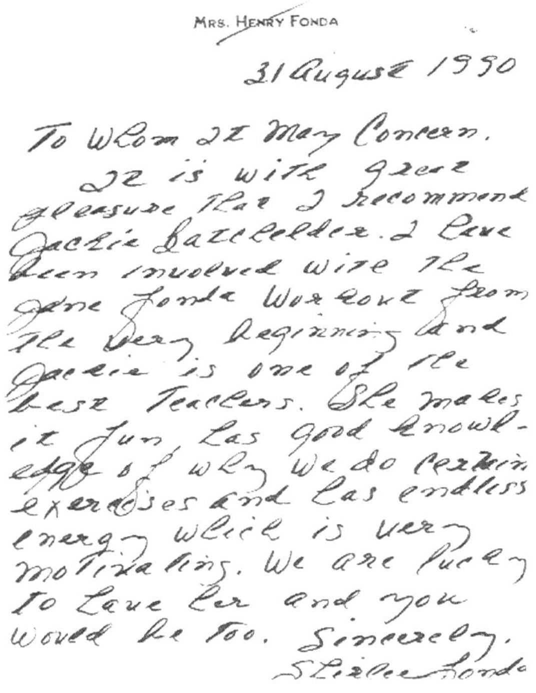

MRS. HENRY FONDA

31 August 1990

To Whom It May Concern.
It is with great
pleasure that I recommend
Jackie Batchelder. I have
been involved with the
Jane Fonda Workout from
the very beginning and
Jackie is one of the
best teachers. She makes
it fun, has good knowl-
edge of why we do certain
exercises and has endless
energy which is very
motivating. We are lucky
to have her and you
would be too. Sincerely,
Shirlee Fonda

Mrs. Henry Fonda a student of mine at Jane Fonda
Workout in Beverly Hills, California.

87

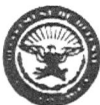

DEPARTMENT OF THE ARMY
United States Army Forces Central Command
Riyadh,Saudi Arabia
APO New York 09852

REPLY TO
ATTENTION OF :

July 10, 1991

TO WHOM IT MAY CONCERN

SUBJECT: Letter Of Recommendation

1. Ms. JACQUELINE BATCHELDER was a member of the SEASPORTS TEAM. Armed Forces Recreation Center in Southwest Asia (SWA) aboard the cruise ship CUNARD PRINCESS from April 10th to July 10th, 1991. Her duties included directing fitness programs, games, and other social activities as part of the rest and relaxation (R&R) program for senior members from all the U.S. military services in SWA.

2. JACQUELINE BATCHELDER was a valued member of our team during her period of employment. She approached all assigned duties in a professional and enthusiastic manner. In superb physical condition herself, she encouraged others who were on R & R to participate in a variety of fitness activities. Her outgoing effervescent personality was a tremendous asset for encouraging others to join in fitness programs. She has a variety of fun games and events, to encourage socialisation among those who were on their three day R & R.

3. JACQUELINE is a natural leader, a mature professional, and a trusted employee. I whole heartedly recommend her for employment in any capacity in recreation programs, fitness programs or public relations activities. She has superb potential for supervisory positions or management in any of the above fields.

In summary, JACQUELINE BATCHELDER has done a superb job for us and I strongly recommend her for employment. She will excel.

MAJOR HENDRICKS
U.S. ARMED FORCES
(AFRC - DESERT STORM)

Major Hendricks from the United States Army during Desert Storm.

Victor Savage,
Hotel Manager,
Cunard Line,
555 Fifth Avenue,
New York,
N. Y. 10017.

9 July 1991

To whom it may concern,

Ref. Ms Jackie Batchelder.

Ms. Batchelder was employed onboard Cunard Princess from April 10th. to July 10th. 1991. She was part of the Seasports team whose function is to promote health and fitness for our current guests. These eclectic activities were extremely well received as Jackie made keeping fit attractive by a unique blend fun and dedication.

The United States Government has chartered the vessel to provide R-and-R for deserving Desert Storm personnel and as such anyone working onboard is subjected to non-stop reveling. This requires patience, tact and a friendly demeanor, which Jackie has shown to the highest level.

She will be missed by all onboard but she will be a great asset to any future employer.

Victor Savage,
Hotel Manager.

Cunard Princess where I provided fitness classes and activities for our Armed Forces during Desert Storm.

12 Week Eating Journal

Week 1	Total Fit Time	Calories Per Day	Lbs. Lost	Reward
Monday				
Tuesday				
Wednesday				
Thursday				
Friday				
Saturday				
Sunday				

Week 2	Total Fit Time	Calories Per Day	Lbs. Lost	Reward
Monday				
Tuesday				
Wednesday				
Thursday				
Friday				
Saturday				
Sunday				

Week 3	Total Fit Time	Calories Per Day	Lbs. Lost	Reward
Monday				
Tuesday				
Wednesday				
Thursday				
Friday				
Saturday				
Sunday				

Week 4	Total Fit Time	Calories Per Day	Lbs. Lost	Reward
Monday				
Tuesday				
Wednesday				
Thursday				
Friday				
Saturday				
Sunday				

Week 5	Total Fit Time	Calories Per Day	Lbs. Lost	Reward
Monday				
Tuesday				
Wednesday				
Thursday				
Friday				
Saturday				
Sunday				

Week 6	Total Fit Time	Calories Per Day	Lbs. Lost	Reward
Monday				
Tuesday				
Wednesday				
Thursday				
Friday				
Saturday				
Sunday				

Week 7	Total Fit Time	Calories Per Day	Lbs. Lost	Reward
Monday				
Tuesday				
Wednesday				
Thursday				
Friday				
Saturday				
Sunday				

Week 8	Total Fit Time	Calories Per Day	Lbs. Lost	Reward
Monday				
Tuesday				
Wednesday				
Thursday				
Friday				
Saturday				
Sunday				

Week 9	Total Fit Time	Calories Per Day	Lbs. Lost	Reward
Monday				
Tuesday				
Wednesday				
Thursday				
Friday				
Saturday				
Sunday				

Week 10	Total Fit Time	Calories Per Day	Lbs. Lost	Reward
Monday				
Tuesday				
Wednesday				
Thursday				
Friday				
Saturday				
Sunday				

Week 11	Total Fit Time	Calories Per Day	Lbs. Lost	Reward
Monday				
Tuesday				
Wednesday				
Thursday				
Friday				
Saturday				
Sunday				

Week 12	Total Fit Time	Calories Per Day	Lbs. Lost	Reward
Monday				
Tuesday				
Wednesday				
Thursday				
Friday				
Saturday				
Sunday				

www.ingramcontent.com/pod-product-compliance
Lightning Source LLC
Chambersburg PA
CBHW022121280326
41933CB00007B/484